The Essential Ketogenic Cookbook

50+ Ketogenic Diet Recipes

DOUGLAS H. MCCALLUM

Table of Contents

Additionally, the information in the following pages is intended only for informational purposes and should thus be thought of as universal. As befitting its nature, it is presented without assurance regarding its prolonged validity or interim quality. Trademarks that are mentioned are done without written consent and can in no way be considered an endorsement from the trademark holder.

Introduction

Congratulations on downloading *The Essential Ketogenic Cookbook: 55 Ketogenic Diet Recipes* and thank you for doing so. Making the decision to switch to a ketogenic lifestyle is a huge step towards looking and feeling healthier than you ever thought possible.

It is only just the first step, however, which is why the following chapters will discuss everything you need to know about the diet, how to ensure you stick with it in the long-term and plenty of recipes to help make sure the transition is as simple and easy as possible. While the ketogenic diet should be suitable for just about everyone, it is important to always discuss any major lifestyle change with a nutritionist or your primary healthcare physician, especially if you have any pre-existing conditions. Failing to do so could ensure you accidentally end up doing more harm than good.

There are plenty of books on this subject on the market, thanks again for choosing this one! Every effort was made to ensure it is full of as much useful information as possible, please enjoy!

Chapter 1:

Understanding the Keto Diet

While there are countless different low-carb diets on the market today, they are all essentially based on the same assumption that there are better ways for the body to burn energy than simply relying completely on carbohydrates. The truth of the matter is that the human body is already ready and willing to burn fat instead of carbohydrates for fuel, it just needs a push in the right direction to start doing so. This process is known as ketosis, but the average American will never experience it as the Standard American Diet is literally overflowing with carbohydrates.

The reason that this is the case is because carbohydrates are much easier to break down into energy than fats are which means that the body will automatically default to using them first whenever possible. With this being made clear, it then follows that in order to switch your body into true fat burning mode all you need to do is to deprive your body of the carbohydrates it is expecting for long enough that you deplete your reserves and give it no other option but to switch to fat burning mode instead.

Prior to the creation of agriculture, humanity existed as hunter gatherers, which meant that there were naturally going to be times when things were somewhat lean. It was to deal with these lean times that the liver developed the ability to use fats to create ketones, which were able to provide the body all of energy it needed. As such, a ketogenic state can be achieved either by cutting out a vast majority of the calories you are consuming, or by tricking your body into thinking this is the case by cutting out a vast majority of the carbohydrates you take in on the regular.

All about ketosis: This means that if you make the decision to swear off carbohydrates then your body will run out of the glucose energy found in carbohydrates and instead start relying on the liver to do its ancestral job. When this happens in your body, the end result is that you will start to look and feel better than you ever thought possible. This in turn brings on what is known as a state of ketosis whereby the liver uses up excess fat (promoting weight loss) to create the energy no longer being provided by the carbohydrates. A Ketogenic/Keto diet changes the body's metabolic pathway from burning glucose for energy to burning fat for energy. When your body burns fats, the results are rapid, but healthy weight loss.

When it comes to the Standard American Diet, most people consume 70 to 80 percent of their daily caloric intake in the form of carbohydrates, 15 to 25 percent in protein and the remainder given over to fats, and not necessarily the healthy kind either. Without access to the healthy fats it needs to function at peak efficiency, the body has no other choice than to generate glucose from the available carbohydrates to power traditional cell function. This glucose is then further broken down into the molecule known as ATP which is the main molecule of energy the body draws from carbohydrates.

This process also creates insulin as a byproduct which is then used to help the ATP get into the bloodstream. Any insulin that is not used up during this task is then used to store excess glucose to ensure it is available for later use as useful, and ultimately forgotten fat. As practically everything you eat is likely full of carbohydrates, there is always stray glucose ready to burn which means the fat stores never get touched, and as a result they continue to grow.

If you are considering the ketogenic diet, then roughly 70 percent of what you eat moving forward should be comprised of healthy fat, with 25 percent dedicated to protein and 5 percent left over for carbohydrates. Those carbohydrates should primarily come from dairy, vegetables or nuts, no starch or wheat allowed. Due to the high amount of naturally occurring foods used in a ketogenic cleanse, the body is able to obtain many vitamins and minerals that are not prevalent in a high carb diet. When the body is consuming sufficient amounts of necessary vitamins and minerals, it is able to heal itself and maintain a healthy immune system. Cleansing your body is one of the best ways to achieve, and maintain, pristine health.

Ketogenic diet versus more traditional diets: To understand what makes the keto diet so very effective, it helps to take a look at a more traditional diet first as the differences will be readily visible. Most diets promote weight loss in a way that is the opposite of how the keto diet works and being prepared for these differences is sure to make your time with the keto diet even more effective.

While the keto diet focuses extensively on the types of foods that you eat, a more traditional diet focuses on limiting calories without spending too much time worrying about just what it is that is accounting for that number. Reducing the the number of calories that you eat in a day will certainly decrease weight gain, but it is really only a temporary solution to a much larger issue. Unlike these diets, the keto diet cuts right to what is really causing the issue and limits you to no more than 15 net grams of carbs per day. The net grams of carbs that are in a given food item can be determined by starting with the total number of carbs and subtracting out any fiber the item might contain. While this will likely be difficult, especially at first, it will be worth it as this will be enough to push the body into a ketogenic state that will cause it to use up its existing fat stores, slimming problem areas and ensuring that new ones never form.

Once you reach a state of ketosis, your body will also begin a secondary process called lipolysis which is used to break down the fat in the body into a pair of molecules, fatty acid and glycerol. The fatty acid is then used directly in the production of ketones as the liver takes it in and produces ketones in response. Ketones are then used for a vast majority of the processes that glucose typically powers; when they aren't enough, such as when the brain needs energy, glycerol is used instead.

Entering ketosis: While this is all well and good, the fact of the matter is that the transition from the Standard American Diet to the ketogenic diet is going to be a rough one, no two ways about it. Your body has spent your entire life refining the ways in which it turns carbohydrates into energy, suddenly cutting off that energy source is going to cause problems, starting with a pronounced lack of energy between the point where you body runs out of available carbs and before the ketone producing systems come online. You should plan for about a week of flu like symptoms, along with the lack of energy, which means you are going to want to pick the right moment if you hope you transition to the ketogenic lifestyle to be truly effective.

This is especially true as, if you give up and give in to your carbohydrate cravings in the short-term, then you will only end up nipping all of your hard work in the bud, as you will have to start all over again if you still hope to reach a state of ketosis. While it may seem like an impossibility at the time, you are also going to want to ensure that you exercise as often as possible during this week, and also skip any extra meals as well. Essentially, any time your stomach rumbles you can count it as another positive step towards ketosis. Finally, you are going to want to try and drink a gallon of water per day as being in ketosis also leads to dehydration.

Alternate Keto diet types: The high protein keto diet is a method used to ease into a Standard Ketogenic Diet when the weight is beyond the normal levels. In this approach, your protein consumption in an SKD is increased by 10 percent and your fat consumption is reduced by 10 percent. This helps those with obesity to help suppress their appetite and reduce their food intake.

The Restricted Ketogenic Diet is a method is not for use by every day otherwise healthy people. It is only worth mentioning it because it has been documented to be used with success for certain brain tumor patients. In this approach, carbohydrate and calorie intake are severely restricted. Because of this the body fully depletes glycogen stores and switches to producing ketones. This method starts with a water fasting regimen and proceeds to only have a Ketogenic Diet of 600 calories a day. After two months or so, ketosis is in full effect and no discernable brain tumor tissue was detected from the tests done.

It is important to keep in mind that this method is absolutely not one to be followed by a person who is in good or fair health. It is only interesting to note because of the effect that glucose and sugar stores have on the brain and the feeding of toxicity in the human body.

Monitoring ketosis: To get your body performing optimally with this method it helps greatly to monitor your ketones and understand where to keep their levels; in order to do this, you will need to buy a ketone meter. You can find these in many different places and in many forms—you can test your blood or your urine. It is highly recommended to use the blood meter due to its accuracy and easy to read results. You can order them online or pick one up from a local pharmacy, prescription-free.

What these strips are testing for is the level of acetone that is currently in your system. The more acetone in your system, the farther into ketosis you are. The most common testing system is via urine strips, but you can also test your level of ketosis naturally by smelling your breath. You will know that you have reached ketosis when your breath begins to smell like a slightly spoiled apple and you can taste a slightly metallic taste on your tongue.

While testing your breath is an easy way to monitor your ongoing ketogenic state, it is recommended that you pick up the urine strips to help you know when you have reached ketosis for the first time. What these strips are testing for is the excess ketones that were not able to be used up normally, and thus end up being flushed from the body as waste. When testing, the magic number is going to be 3, anything lower than this and your body is still adapting to the keto lifestyle. If your ketones continue increasing past 3 then you are going to want to increase the amount of calories you are consuming per day as this is a sign that your body is getting all the nutrients it needs.

Ketogenic benefits: While getting there is certainly not easy, once you enter a ketogenic state you will find that your new state provides a wide variety of health benefits outside of simple weight loss. This diet has shown evidence that it can reduce the episodes of epileptic seizures in adults as well as children, even when a less strict form of the diet is used. The results of current research studies suggest that the ketogenic diet protects neurons and modifies diseases for many adults who have neurodegenerative disorders. Other benefits of the ketogenic diet are increased energy, improved performance, mental clarity, improved cognitive function, better digestion, and a slowdown of the aging process.

The keto diet has also been proven to help combat a wide variety of diseases, including many common types of cancer. Many cancer cell types are known to feed on glucose, in much the same way that normal cells do. Unlike more traditional cells, however, the mutated cells are unable to survive purely on ketones which means that without glucose they will grow much more slowly than they otherwise would. Decreasing the amount of carbs consumed on the regular also decrease the amount of gluten that is regularly consumed, as an estimated 30 percent of the population has an untreated gluten allergy, the benefits you experience could be surprising.

Finally, it is also known to help combat Alzheimer's disease as well as dementia, two problems that are thought to coincide with a buildup of glucose tolerance. While the brain needs glucose to live, a prolonged exposure to extremely high levels can cause a buildup of the brain's tolerance towards insulin. This, in turn, makes it more difficult for the brain to take in the glucose that it needs in order for it to continue functioning at its ideal levels. As ketosis provides a healthy alternative for the brain to receive all the fuel it needs, without any of the risks, experts believe that it will see increased use in combating these and other similar issues.

Chapter 2:

All About Macros

To understand how Ketosis works, you must first understand how your body turns the food that you eat into energy, and how your body uses this energy. I am sure you remember learning in second-grade science class that the food you eat is converted into energy during the digestive process. What you might not remember, however, is how exactly your body sources the energy it needs from these foods.

Digestion is the mechanism whereby your body goes about breaking down food through mechanical and chemical processes. Without segmenting food into their simpler forms, your body cannot use it for energy, growth, and cell repair.

The food that you eat consists of nutrients that can be primarily divided into two classifications: macronutrients and micronutrients.

Micronutrients are the vast array of vitamins and minerals needed to assist your body in repair, growth, and protecting itself. Micronutrients cannot be found naturally occurring in the body, and so they must come from your diet. While they are vital for the proper functioning of your body, they are only required in small amounts.

You acquire macronutrients from the fats, carbohydrates, and protein you eat. Each macronutrient serves a specific purpose in your body, but their main purpose is to provide the energy your body needs. Because of this, your body needs a relatively large quantity of macronutrients to satisfy the demands of its functioning systems.

Carbohydrates

Carbohydrates come from the sugars, starches, and fiber found in the fruits, grains, and vegetables that you eat. Through the digestive process, these carbohydrates are broken down by natural chemicals in your mouth, small intestine, and pancreas.

In the mouth, your chewing breaks down the food you eat into smaller chunks, and your saliva mixes with it and begins to break it down so that it will be more easily digested by your body. After passing through your stomach, the food enters your small intestine where it will be mixed with enzymes that were released by the pancreas, and bile sent by the liver. The micronutrients and macronutrients from the food you ate will be absorbed into your bloodstream as the food passes through your small intestine. This process helps to break down the carbohydrates into glucose, sucrose, and fructose. These are the simple sugars your body utilizes for its immediate energy needs.

During this digestive process, your pancreas has been busy secreting a hormone called insulin. The insulin's purpose is to help carry the glucose into your body's cells when they need energy. Glucose cannot enter your energy-starved cells on its own, it needs help. The insulin is like a toll bridge, allowing the glucose to gain passage into the cell where it is quickly converted into energy.

Remember the nutrients were absorbed into the bloodstream via the small intestine during this process, and they are now looking for a job to do. The glucose will travel to the liver, where it will be further broken down into other chemicals your body needs. One of these chemicals is glycogen. Your body can store only a limited amount of glycogen, about 100 grams in the liver and 500 grams in the muscles. Once those storage tanks are full, your body must determine what to do with the rest of the glycogen it produced from the carbs you ate. Your liver will go through a process that will convert the excess glycogen into fatty acids which it will send back out into the body via the bloodstream. These fatty acids will be stored throughout your body in fat cells.

Protein

Protein is one of the macronutrients your body will need in decent quantities. Protein is a crucial element involved in almost all of your body's biological processes. Your protein sources will come from meat, eggs, soy, and beans that you eat. These foods are all broken down and digested in the stomach, small intestines, and pancreas. As a result, the protein is broken down into its core component, the amino acid, to make it much easier for the body to . These are used by your body to create neurotransmitters, non-essential amino acids and other protein-based compounds in your body.

Overall, there are 20 amino acids that are crucial to a well-functioning body, only 10 of which your body can produce on its own. The rest must come from the food you eat. The body is unable to store excess amino acids to use when later necessary. Instead, each day the amino acids must be created by the digestion of protein. If you do consume too much protein your body will absorb the amino acids into the bloodstream through the small intestine. The excess amino acids will be transported to the liver where they will be chemically altered into ammonia. As ammonia is highly toxic if allowed to accumulate in our body, it will be sent back through the bloodstream to the kidneys, and on to the bladder to be excreted.

I would like to note one exception though. The human body is an amazing machine and is capable of incredible things. One of these feats is that if your glucose stores dip too low, your liver will embark on a process known as gluconeogenesis. What this means is that your liver can actually convert some of the amino acids into glucose. Protein is not your body's first choice when hunting for energy (in fact, it is your body's last resort), but it does have the ability to make this conversion when absolutely necessary to sustain life.

Fats

Fat is another macronutrient source your body needs. You will ingest fats from the oils, seeds, nuts, and fat in your diet. Again, only some of the necessary fatty acids can be produced by systems in your body. The others must be introduced to your body through your diet.

The fat you eat will go through the same digestive process that carbohydrates and protein do. As it makes its way through the small intestine, the gallbladder is hailed to send a supply of bile while digestive enzymes are ordered from the pancreas. These will help the fat to be broken down into two useful components, glycerol and fatty acids.

The glycerol and fatty acids will be absorbed into the cells lining the wall of the small intestine. Here, fats are different from the other macronutrients. Because the fat molecules are too large to pass through the capillaries, they are instead absorbed into the lymphatic system. When the lymphatic system collides with the veins, this is when the fat molecules will finally make it into the bloodstream.

Once there, they will be used for a wide variety of different, crucial, bodily processes including the repair of cells and the creation of new tissue. Fatty acids are sometimes stored as fat cells. Other times, after fat cells, have gone through the digestive process and been converted into fatty acids; they can be sent to haul fats and cholesterol through your bloodstream. The fatty acids are also used by your body to regulate your temperature. When mixed with oxygen, water, and carbon dioxide; the fat is excreted from your body in sweat, or breathed out of your lungs.

Vitamins

Vitamins are in the micronutrient group, along with minerals. These substances come from the food solids and liquid that you eat. As with everything else you consume, these substances are broken down by your system through the digestive process. As they pass through the small and large intestines, your body will absorb the vitamins. These different vitamins are a necessity for use in different body functions. Vitamins and minerals are crucial ingredients needed for everything from fighting inflammation to repairing cell damage.

More on Digestion

Everything you eat will be absorbed in your small intestines by specialized cells that pass across the intestinal lining. Your bloodstream circulates the salts, vitamins, glycerol, amino acids and required sugars to your liver. Your liver processes everything you feed to your body and puts it all to work to keep you performing as best as you can. The vast network that connects all of your blood vessels together is known as the lymphatic system and its job is to move lymph, along with your white blood cells wherever they need to be. Vital compounds are circulated throughout your body via the lymph system. Eventually, your lymph system connects to your circulatory system, and the micronutrients carried by it enter into your bloodstream.

The whole process of digestion is controlled by your nervous system and the hormones and digestive enzymes your body produces. These hormones and enzymes are created from every organ involved in the digestive process. I explained that bile is an enzyme produced by the liver and stored in the gallbladder. Bile is a necessary ingredient in helping to digest the fats and fat-soluble vitamins you consume. Insulin is a hormone secreted by the pancreas, and it is paramount to your body's cells being able to use glucose for energy. Insulin is also necessary to regulate the level of sugar in your blood.

Your digestive system has its own nervous system that operates separately from your main nervous system. The digestive nervous system is called the enteric nervous system. This system is massive. It is contained within the walls of your entire digestive system, extending from the esophagus all the way to the anus. It also boasts the same number of neurons as your spinal cord. The enteric nervous system is involved in the creation of neurotransmitters, which are the chemicals your brain uses to send information through your body. Some of the neurotransmitters created by the enteric nervous system function solely to aid in digestion. So, we see the system come full circle. The food you eat enables your body to produce the necessary chemicals to create neurotransmitters, while the neurotransmitters created to aid in the digestion of the food you eat.

While the enteric nervous system can operate autonomously, it must communicate with the central nervous system to properly do its job. The two systems are connected by fibers in the digestive pathway. The systems can interact through these fibers, sending messages that force the other system to carry out necessary tasks. Because of this connection, your digestive system can also be controlled by outside influences. Delicious smelling food can cause your mouth to start producing saliva, which is one of the first contributors to the digestive process. Even just seeing the food you think looks good will start these processes. Your tempted eyes will send information to your brain which will send messages to your stomach via neurotransmitters; then your stomach will start secreting the acids necessary for breaking down the food your body thinks it is about to receive.

In the digestive process, the nerves in this system cause the muscles of your gastrointestinal tract to contract or relax in order to digest food. This process provides for the release of substances to control the way digestive enzymes and food move. Your hormones, on the other hand, regulate appetite and stimulate the production of digestive juices.

You have already learned of hormones involved in digestion (such as insulin), but are you aware that there are certain hormones in your body that serve only one purpose-to make you control your hunger? Leptin and ghrelin are the names of these hormones. Leptin is created by fat cells, and the purpose of this hormone is to decrease your appetite and let your body know when it has had its fill. Ghrelin is the hormone responsible for increasing your appetite and letting your body know when it is hungry.

After your body completes the digestive process and has taken everything it needs from the food you have given it, there will be excess nutrients that your body will not need. The excess glycogen will be stored in your liver, muscle, and fat cells. Leftover fat is converted into triglycerides that is then stored within fat cells. Excess amino acids are excreted through urine. Leftover vitamins and minerals are either expelled through urine, if water-soluble, or stored in the liver and fat cells, if fat soluble.

Examples of the breakdown of common foods

Proteins

- Chicken wings (4 oz / 250 cal / 18g fat / 0g net carbs / 21g protein)

- Salmon (4 oz / 236 cal / 15g fat / 0g net carbs / 23g protein)

- Lobster (4 oz / 114 cal / .68g fat / 1g net carbs / 24g protein)

- Sardines (1 can / 191 cal / 11g fat / 0g net carbs / 23g protein)

- Tuna (1 packet / 70 cal / .5g fat / 0g net carbs / 17g protein)

- Ground lamb (4 oz / 319 cal / 27g fat / 0g net carbs / 19g protein)

- Liver (4 oz / 135 cal / 5g fat / 0g net carbs / 19g protein)

- Ground bison (4 oz / 190 cal / 11g fat / 0g net carbs / 23g protein)

- Deer (4 oz / 130 cal / 2g fat / 0g net carbs / 26g protein)

- Egg (1 large / 70 cal / 5g fat / 0.5g net carbs / 6g protein)

- Almond butter (2 tbsp / 180 cal / 16g fat / 4g net carbs / 6g protein)

Dairy

- Mascarpone (1 oz. / 120 cal / 13g fat / 0g net carbs / 2g protein)

- Mozzarella (1 oz. / 70 cal / 5g fat / 1g net carbs / 5g protein)

- Brie (1 oz. / 95 cal / 8g fat / 0g net carbs / 6g protein)

- Aged Cheddar (1 oz. / 110 cal / 9g fat / 0g net carbs / 7g protein)

- Parmesan (1 oz. / 110 cal / 7g fat / 1g net carbs / 10g protein)

Fruits/veggies

- Green Beans (6 oz. / 26 cal / 0g fat / 4g net carbs / 2g protein)

- Yellow Onion (6 oz. / 68 cal / 0g fat / 12g net carbs / 2g protein)

- Blackberries (6 oz. / 73 cal / 1g fat / 8g net carbs / 2g protein)

- Raspberries (6 oz. / 88 cal / 1g fat / 8g net carbs / 2g protein)

- Cherries (1 C / .5g fat / 16g net carbs / 2g protein)

- Pears (1 med / 102 cal / 0g fat / 21g net carbs / .5g protein)

- Raspberries (1 C / 65 cal / 1g fat / 7g net carbs / 1.5g protein)

- Blackberries (1 C / 62 cal / 1g fat / 6g net carbs / 2g protein)

- Watermelon (1 wedge / 87 cal / .5g fat / 21g net carbs / 2g protein)

Chapter 3:

Breakfast Recipes

Avocado smoothie

This recipe needs 5 minutes to prepare, 0 minutes to cook and will make 1 serving.

- Net Carbs: 6 grams

- Protein: 26 grams

- Fats: 38 grams

- Calories: 587

What to Use

- Cacao nibs (1.5 T)

- Ice (5 cubes)

- Coconut oil (2 T)

- Stevia (to taste)

- Gelatin (.5 T)

- Whey protein powder (1 scoop)

- Chia seeds (1 T)

- Avocado (.5)

- Unsweetened coconut milk (1 c)

What to Do

- For a thicker smoothie, prepare the night before by combining the coconut milk and the chia seeds together and mix well. Stir several times over 2 or 3 hours and then let it thicken overnight.

- When you are ready to drink your smoothie, slice the avocado lengthwise before removing the seeds and the skin. Add the sliced avocado, along with the remaining ingredients, except the ice and coconut oil to your blender and blend well.

- Add in the liquid coconut oil and incorporate thoroughly. Keeping this step separate from adding the ice keeps the smoothie nice and smooth.

- Add in the ice and blend until it reaches your desired level of thickness.

Green Smoothie

This recipe needs 5 minutes to prepare, 0 minutes to cook and will make 6 servings (1 cup each).

- Protein: 18 grams

- Net Carbs: 3 grams

- Fats: 26.4 grams

- Calories: 337

What to Use

- Stevia (as desired)

- Avocado (.5)

- Kiwi (.5 c chopped, peeled)

- Cucumber (1 c sliced, peeled)

- Ginger (1 T chopped, peeled)

- Parsley (2 T)

- Pineapple (.3 c chopped)

- Lettuce (1 c)

- Ice cubes (5)

- Coconut oil (2 T)

- Chia seeds (1 T)

- Vanilla whey protein powder (1 scoop)

What to Do

- Slice the avocado lengthwise before removing the seeds and the skin. Add the sliced avocado, along with the remaining ingredients to your blender and blend well.

- Add in the liquid coconut oil and incorporate thoroughly. Keeping this step separate from adding the ice keeps the smoothie nice and smooth

- Add in the ice and blend until it reaches your desired thickness.

Beet breakfast smoothie

This recipe needs 3 minutes to prepare, 10 minutes to cook and will make 2 servings.

- Protein: 14.7 grams

- Net Carbs: 6.2 grams

- Fats: 42.4 grams

- Calories: 420

What to Use

- Stevia (to taste)

- Vanilla (.25 tsp.)

- Cacao powder (3 T)

- Beet (1)

- Avocado (.5)

- Ice (5 cubes)

- Coconut milk (2 c)

- Coconut oil (2 T)

What to Do

- Place the beet in a small pot and fill the pot with water before placing it on the stove over a burner turned to a high heat. Once the water boils, turn the heat down and let the beet simmer, covered for 10 minutes.

- Slice the avocado lengthwise before removing the seeds and the skin. Add the sliced avocado, along with the remaining ingredients, except the ice and coconut oil to your blender and blend well.

- Add in the liquid coconut oil and incorporate thoroughly. Keeping this step separate from adding the ice keeps the smoothie nice and smooth.

- Add in the ice and blend until it reaches your desired level of thickness

Strawberry smoothie

This recipe needs 5 minutes to prepare, 0 minutes to cook and will make 1 serving.

- Protein: 27 grams

- Net Carbs: 5.4 grams

- Fats: 25.6 grams

- Calories: 312

What to Use

- Chia seeds (1 T)

- Almonds (2 T)

- Cinnamon (.5 tsp.)

- Strawberries (.5 c frozen)

- Coconut milk (1 c)

What to Do

- For a thicker smoothie, prepare the night before by combining the coconut milk and the chia seeds together and mix well. Stir several times over 2 or 3 hours and then let it thicken overnight.

- When you are ready to drink, add all of the ingredients to your blender and blend until it reaches your desired consistency.

Shakshouka

This recipe needs 10 minutes to prepare, 35 minutes to cook and will make 4 servings.

- Protein: 26.1 grams

- Net Carbs: 4.5 grams

- Fats: 41.6 grams

- Calories: 571

What to Use

- Eggs (5)

- Pepper (as desired)

- Salt (as desired)

- Chili powder (.25 tsp.)

- Paprika (1 tsp.)

- Cumin powder (1 tsp.)

- Tomatoes (1.5 chopped)

- Bell pepper (.5 chopped)

- Serrano pepper (.25 chopped)

- Garlic (1.5 cloves chopped)

- White onion (.5 chopped)

- Ghee (2 T)

What to Do

- Add the ghee to a skillet before placing it on the stove over a medium heat and adding in the onion. Let it cook for approximately 10 minutes, stirring consistently until it begins to soften.

- Add in the serrano pepper along with the garlic and let them cook for 2 minutes before adding in the red bell pepper and turning the heat to low. Let all the ingredients cook an additional 10 minutes, stirring consistently.

- Mix in the tomatoes and the remaining spices before letting the dish simmer and continue cooking until the sauce has reduced to your desired level.

- Add the eggs to the skillet before seasoning as desired and letting everything cook, covered for approximately 5 minutes until the eggs reach your desired level of doneness

Breakfast keto pizza

This recipe needs 10 minutes to prepare, 35 minutes to cook and will make 6 servings.

- Protein: 19.2 grams

- Net Carbs: 5.8 grams

- Fats: 34.5 grams

- Calories: 360

What to Use - Crust

- Baking soda (.5 tsp.)

- Italian seasoning (2 tsp.)

- Garlic powder (2 tsp.)

- Onion powder (1 tsp.)

- Unsweetened coconut milk (1 c)

- Coconut flour (.5 c)

- Egg whites (6)

What to Use -Toppings

- Extra virgin olive oil (1 T)

- Red pepper flakes (.5 tsp.)

- Baby spinach (3 c)

- Tomato (.5 sliced thin)

- Eggs (3)

What to Do

- Start by making sure your oven is heated to 375F.

- Using parchment paper, cover a large baking sheet)

- Combine the coconut milk, seasonings and egg whites in a mixing bowl and whisk well before adding in coconut flour and combining thoroughly.

- Spread the dough onto the baking sheet evenly before placing the baking sheet in the oven for approximately 16 minutes.

- Once the crust has finished cooking, turn the oven temp to 350F.

- Spread the olive oil evenly across the crust before topping with spinach, tomato and egg before topping with red pepper.

- Place the baking sheet back into the oven for approximately 12 minutes or the eggs have fully set.

Keto scramble

This recipe needs 10 minutes to prepare, 10 minutes to cook and will make 1 serving.

- Protein: 21 grams

- Net Carbs: 5 grams

- Fats: 29 grams

- Calories: 350

What to Use

- Pepper (as desired)

- Salt (as desired)

- Deli ham (2 slices)

- Spinach (.5 c)

- Red bell pepper (.25 c)

- Baby Bella mushrooms (4)

- Eggs (3 whisked)

- Ghee (1 T divided)

What to Do

- Chop the ham and the vegetables and mix well.

- Add the ghee to a frying pan before placing the pan on top of a burner turned to a high/medium heat. Add in the ham and vegetables and sauté.

- In a second frying pan, add the rest of ghee and place it on a burner turned to a medium heat. After it melts, add in the eggs and let them cook, stirring regularly to prevent burning. Season as desired.

- Combine the two skillets and serve.

Spinach and Sausage Frittata

This recipe needs 15 minutes to prepare, 30 minutes to cook and will make 9 servings (2 muffins per serving).

- Protein: 16 grams

- Net Carbs: 2 grams

- Fats: 20 grams

- Calories: 274

What to Use

- Nutmeg (.25 tsp. ground)

- Pepper (as desired)

- Salt (as desired)

- Unsweetened almond milk (.5 c plain)

- Heavy cream (.5 c)

- Eggs (12)

- Feta cheese (.5 c)

- Spinach (10 oz. frozen, chopped, thawed, drained)

- Breakfast sausage (12 oz.)

What to Do

- Ensure your oven is heated to 375F

- Grease 18 muffin cups

- Crumble the sausage into pieces in a mixing bowl.

- Ensure all of the liquid is removed from the spinach before adding it to the bowl with the sausage and mixing well.

- Add in the feta cheese and toss lightly until combined before adding the results to the greased muffin cups.

- In a large bowl, combine the nutmeg, pepper, salt, almond milk, cream and eggs and then add the results to the muffin cups until they are roughly 75 percent full.

- Add the muffin tins to the oven and let them bake for half an hour or until they are fully set.

- Let cool 5 minutes prior to serving.

Breakfast skillet

This recipe needs 5 minutes to prepare, 5 minutes to cook and will make 4 serving.

- Protein: 35.4 grams

- Net Carbs: 4.25 grams

- Fats: 41.8 grams

- Calories: 578

What to Use

- Coconut oil (1 T)

- Dijon mustard (2 T)

- Basil (.5 tsp.)

- Salt (.5 tsp.)

- Garlic powder (.5 tsp.)

- Pepper (.5 tsp.)

- Zucchini (2 trimmed, sliced)

- Mushrooms (8 oz. chopped coarse)

- Pork (1 lb. ground)

What to Do

- Add 1 T coconut oil to a skillet before placing it on the stove over a burner turned to a high/medium heat. Add the mushrooms to the skillet and allow them to cook for 3 minutes before adding in the zucchini and seasoning as desired. Let everything cook for an additional 3 minutes.

- Spread the vegetables to the side of the pan, before adding in the pork to the open space and seasoning as desired. Let the meat cook fully before mixing the ingredients together.

- Mix in the Dijon mustard and let everything cook an additional 60 seconds prior to serving.

Breakfast sausage with blueberries

This recipe needs 5 minutes to prepare, 10 minutes to cook and will make 8 servings (2 patties per serving).

- Protein: 10 grams

- Net Carbs: 1 grams

- Fats: 12 grams

- Calories: 110

What to Use

- Coconut oil (2 T)

- Pepper (as desired)

- Salt (as desired)

- Blackberries (.5 c frozen, halved)

- Garlic powder (.5 tsp.)

- Thyme (.5 tsp. dried)

- Sage (.5 tsp. dried, ground)

- Pork (1 lb. ground)

What to Do

- Add all of the ingredients, save the coconut oil and blackberries to a large mixing bowl and combine thoroughly.

- Shape the results into 16 1 oz. patties before adding in the blackberries.

- Add the coconut oil to the skillet before placing it on a burner turned to a medium heat and letting it melt before adding in the patties a few at a time. Each patty should only need to cook about 2 minutes per side.

- Uneaten servings can be stored for up to 4 days in the refrigerator.

Chorizo Casserole

This recipe needs 15 minutes to prepare, 45 minutes to cook and will make 4 servings.

- Protein: 35.7 grams

- Net Carbs: 6.2 grams

- Fats: 44.9 grams

- Calories: 579

What to Use

- Green onion (.5 diced)

- Pepper (as desired)

- Salt (as desired)

- Eggs (4 whisked)

- Garlic powder (.5 tsp.)

- Cauliflower (1 small head, florets)

- Green chilis (12 oz. diced)

- Yellow onion (.5 diced)

- Chorizo (1 lb.)

What to Do

- Start by making sure your oven is heated to 375F.

- Place a large skillet on top of a burner turned to a medium heat before adding in the onion and chorizo and letting the chorizo brown.

- After the meat has finished cooking, add in the chilies and combine thoroughly before removing the skillet from the stove and adding the results to a large bowl.

- Use a food processor to puree the cauliflower to create cauliflower rice.

- Add the cauliflower rice to the mixing bowl before mixing in the egg and any seasonings and combining thoroughly.

- Add everything to a greased baking dish (9x13) and put it in the oven for 45 minutes.

- Let cool 5 minutes prior to serving.

Chapter 4:

Lunch Recipes

Keto meatballs

This recipe needs 10 minutes to prepare, 30 minutes to cook and will make 9 meatballs.

- Protein: 12 grams

- Net Carbs: 2 grams

- Fats: 7 grams

- Calories: 89

What to Use

- Coconut oil (2 T)

- Pepper (as desired)

- Salt (as desired)

- Oregano (1 T)

- White onion (2 T diced)

- Garlic (2 T minced)

- Bacon (9 slices)

- Italian sausage (1 lb.)

What to Do

- Start by making sure your oven is heated to 375F.

- Cover a baking sheet using aluminum foil.

- Place a skillet on top of a burner that has been turned to a high/medium heat before adding in the coconut oil and the sausage and letting it brown.

- Add all of the ingredients, save the bacon to a mixing bowl and combine thoroughly.

- Form the results into 9 meatballs and wrap a slice of bacon around each before placing them on the baking sheet. Place the baking sheet in the oven for 30 minutes or until the bacon is well-cooked.

- Let cool 5 minutes prior to serving.

Salami and cream cheese pinwheels

This recipe needs 15 minutes to prepare, 30 minutes to cook and will make 5 servings (4 pinwheels per serving).

- Protein: 16.7 grams

- Net Carbs: 1.2 grams

- Fats: 16.8 grams

- Calories: 6200

What to Use

- Pepper (as desired)

- Salt (as desired)

- Pickles (4 T)

- Salami (10 slices)

- Cream cheese (8 oz.)

What to Do

- Leave the cream cheese out until it reaches room temperature before placing it in a bowl and whipping it well.

- Spread the results onto a piece of plastic wrap so that it forms a .25-inch-thick square.

- Top the cream cheese with the pickles before topping the pickles with the salami in overlapping pieces.

- Place another layer of plastic wrap on the salami and press down firmly before flipping the entire thing over and peeling back the top plastic wrap layer from the cream cheese.

- Slowly roll the rectangle into a log shape, removing the plastic wrap as you go.

- Slice the log and serve.

Bratwurst wrapped in bacon

This recipe needs 5 minutes to prepare, 20 minutes to cook and will make 4 servings.

- Protein:28 grams

- Net Carbs: 2.6 grams

- Fats: 34 grams

- Calories: 507

What to Use

- Bratwurst (4)

- Pepper (as desired)

- Salt (as desired)

- Cheese (4 slices)

- Romaine lettuce (4 leaves)

- Bacon (4 slices)

- Beer (24 oz.)

What to Do

- Add the beer to a pan before adding in the bratwurst and placing it on top of a burner turned to a high heat. Let them cook, covered for 10 minutes.

- Remove the bratwurst from the pan and wrap each in bacon.

- Place the bratwurst on a preheated grill and grill until the bacon is crispy.

- Wrap in a piece of lettuce prior to serving.

Spicy Thai Chicken

This recipe needs 7 minutes to prepare, 8 minutes to cook and will make 4 servings.

- Protein: 25 grams

- Net Carbs: 5.1 grams

- Fats: 31.6 grams

- Calories: 298

What to Use

- Coconut oil (2 T)

- Pepper (as desired)

- Salt (as desired)

- Basil (3 T chopped)

- Hoisin sauce (.25 c)

- Coleslaw mix (.25 c)

- Green onions (.5 chopped)

- Red bell pepper (.25 sliced thin)

- Garlic (4 cloves minced)

- Ginger (1 T minced)

- Red curry paste (2 T)

- Chicken (1 lb. ground)

What to Do

- Add the coconut oil to a skillet before placing it on the stove over a burner turned to a high heat. Add in the chicken and let it brown before breaking it up with the help of a wooden spoon.

- Mix in the red curry paste, coleslaw, peppers and garlic and let everything cook for 3 minutes before adding in the green onions and hoisin sauce and tossing well.

- Remove the skillet from the burner, add the basil and toss.

Salmon with mushrooms and bok choy

This recipe needs 10 minutes to prepare, 20 minutes to cook and will make 4 servings.

- Protein: 20.6 grams

- Net Carbs: 4.1 grams

- Fats: 35 grams

- Calories: 527

What to Use

- Coconut oil (2 T)

- Pepper (as desired)

- Salt (as desired)

- Lemon juice (.5 lemon)

- Ginger (.5 in. grated)

- Coconut aminos (1 T)

- Sesame oil (1 tsp.)

- Green onion (.5)

- Sesame seeds (1 T toasted)

- Bok choy (4)

- Portobello mushroom (2 caps)

- Salmon fillet (4)

What to Do

- Combine .5 tsp. pepper, .5 tsp. salt, lemon juice, ginger, coconut aminos, sesame oil and the coconut oil together in a mixing bowl and whisk well.

- Add half of the marinade to the salmon and coat thoroughly. Cover the fish and let it sit, refrigerated for at least 60 minutes to give the fish time to marinate.

- Ensure your oven is heated to 400F.

- Trim the bok choy and cut it in half, slice the mushrooms to they are in .5-inch pieces before topping with the remaining marinade, tossing well, and placing onto a prepared baking sheet, leave room for the salmon.

- Add the salmon to the baking sheet, skin down, and place the baking sheet in the oven for approximately 20 minutes until the fish flakes easily when you touch it with a fork.

Avocado stuffed with bacon and chicken

This recipe needs 10 minutes to prepare, 20 minutes to cook and will make 3 servings.

- Protein: 22 grams

- Net Carbs: 2.2 grams

- Fats: 31 grams

- Calories: 326

What to Use

- Keto mayo (.3 c)

- Pepper (as desired)

- Salt (as desired)

- Grape tomatoes (.3 c chopped)

- Avocado (2)

- Bacon (3 pieces chopped, cooked)

- Chicken breasts (2 cubed)

What to Do

- Place the chicken in a bowl and season well before placing it, and the bacon on the grill.

- Add all of the ingredients, except the avocado to a bowl and mix well.

- Cut the avocados in half, remove the pit and fill each half with the chicken mixture.

Enchilada bowl

This recipe needs 10 minutes to prepare, 10 minutes to cook and will make 4 servings.

- Protein: 18 grams

- Net Carbs: 5.1 grams

- Fats: 22 grams

- Calories: 240

What to Use

- Coconut oil (2 T)

- Pepper (as desired)

- Salt (as desired)

- Avocado (1 chopped)

- Cauliflower rice (12 oz.)

- Green chilies (4 oz.)

- Onion (.25 c)

- Water (.25 c)

- Enchilada sauce (.75 c red sauce)

- Chicken breasts (2, cut into 4 pieces each)

What to Do

- Add the coconut oil to the skillet before placing it on the stove on top of a burner turned to a medium heat.

- Add in the water, onion, chilies and enchilada sauce before reducing the heat and letting it simmer, covered until the chicken reaches an internal temperature of 165F.

- Once the chicken is cooked, shred it and add it back into the sauce and let it simmer for another 10 minutes, this time uncovered.

- Plate the chicken with the rice and the chopped avocado.

Tuna salad with avocado

This recipe needs 10 minutes to prepare, 10 minutes to cook and will make 4 servings.

- Protein: 15.6 grams

- Net Carbs: 4.2 grams

- Fats: 21.5 grams

- Calories: 266

What to Use

- Coconut oil (2 T)

- Pepper (as desired)

- Salt (as desired)

- Lemon juice (2 T)

- Cilantro (.25 c chopped)

- Red onion (1 small, sliced thin)

- Avocados (2 large, sliced, pitted, peeled)

- Cucumber (1 sliced)

- Tuna (15 oz., flaked, drained)

What to Do

- Combine all of the ingredients save the oil and lemon juice together in a salad bowl and toss.

- In a small bowl, combine .25 tsp. pepper, 1 tsp. salt, 2 T coconut oil and 2 T lemon juice and mix well.

- Top salad with dressing prior to serving and mix well.

Chicken and Brussels Sprouts

This recipe needs 10 minutes to prepare, 25 minutes to cook and will make 2 servings.

- Protein: 16 grams

- Net Carbs: 4 grams

- Fats: 28.6 grams

- Calories: 564

What to Use

- Coconut oil (2 T)

- Pepper (as desired)

- Salt (as desired)

- Thyme (1 tsp.)

- Lemon juice (1 T)

- Spicy mustard (.25 c)

- Chicken breast (2)

- Brussels sprouts (.5 lb. sliced)

What to Do

- Add the thyme, lemon juice, spicy mustard and seasonings to a small ramekin and whisk well to combine.

- Add the chicken breasts to a bowl and top with the mustard, ensuring the chicken is well coated. Place the bowl, covered, into the refrigerator and let it marinate, for at least 60 minutes.

- Ensure your oven is heated to 350F.

- Prepare a baking sheet by covering it using parchment paper.

- Set the sliced brussels sprouts into a bowl before adding in the coconut oil and salt and pepper as needed before tossing well.

- Place the brussels sprouts on the baking sheet so they form a single layer.

- Add the chicken to a glass baking pan before placing the baking pan in the oven for 10 minutes. At that point add the baking sheet to the oven as well and let everything cook an additional 15 minutes.

Asparagus and Lemon Chicken

This recipe needs 5 minutes to prepare, 25 minutes to cook and will make 4 servings.

- Protein: 12 grams

- Net Carbs: 5 grams

- Fats: 18.7 grams

- Calories: 183

What to Use

- Coconut oil (2 T divided)

- Pepper (as desired)

- Salt (as desired)

- Chicken stock (1 c)

- Dijon mustard (1 T)

- Lemon zest (.5 lemon)

- Lemon juice (3 T)

- Garlic (2 cloves crushed)

- Asparagus stalks (1 lb.)

- Tapioca flour (.25 c)

- Chicken breast (4 skinless, boneless)

What to Do

- Start by placing each of the chicken breasts between a pair of pieces of plastic wrap before pounding them down until they are about .25 inches thick each.

- Add the pepper, salt and flour to a mixing bowl before adding in the chicken and ensuring it is well coated.

- Add 1 T of the oil to a skillet before placing it on top of a burner turned to a high/medium heat. Once the oil is thoroughly heated, add in the chicken and let it cook approximately 5 minutes per side or until it reaches an internal temperature of at least 165 degrees. Remove it from the skillet while you cook the asparagus.

- Add the rest of the oil to the skillet before adding in the asparagus stalks and letting them cook for 60 seconds before adding in the garlic and letting it cook for yet another minute.

- While it is cooking, mix together the mustard and lemon juice in a small cup and whisk well. Add the results to the skill and turn the heat up to allow the liquid to boil.

- Once it does so, reduce the heat and allow it to boil for approximately 3 minutes until the asparagus becomes tender.

- Plate the chicken and top with the asparagus and the excess liquid.

Lasagna with Zoodles

This recipe needs 15 minutes to prepare, 30 minutes to cook and will make 4 servings.

- Protein: 34 grams

- Net Carbs: 4 grams

- Fats: 41 grams

- Calories: 544

What to Use

- Mozzarella cheese (4 oz.)

- Ricotta cheese (10 oz.)

- Zucchini (1 large)

- Low carb marinara sauce (1 c)

- Ground beef (16 oz.)

What to Do

- Start by making sure your oven is heated to 350F.

- Peel the zucchini so it forms strips, taking care to avoid the seeds at the core. Salt the result and leave them be for 15 minutes before pressing them with paper towels to remove excess moisture.

- Add the ground beef to a skillet and place it on top of a burner turned to a high/medium heat. Add in the marinara and season as desired.

- Add the meat to a small casserole dish starting with the meet, then zoodles, then cheese and repeat so that cheese ends up on top.

- Cover the casserole dish using tin foil and place it in the oven for 30 minutes.

- Broil an additional 3 minutes to brown the cheese on top and let sit 5 minutes prior to serving.

Pizza Chicken

This recipe needs 15 minutes to prepare, 30 minutes to cook and will make 6 servings.

- Protein: 25 grams

- Net Carbs: 6 grams

- Fats: 38 grams

- Calories: 492

What to Use

- Broccoli (2 c steamed)

- Pepperoni (2 oz.)

- Mozzarella cheese (4 oz.)

- Pizza seasoning (1.5 T)

- Pizza sauce (.5 c)

- Chicken breast (1 lb.)

What to Do

- Start by making sure your oven is heated to 375F.

- Add the chicken to a baking sheet, top with pizza seasoning and pizza sauce before placing the baking sheet in the oven for 8 minutes.

- Remove the baking sheet from the oven, top the chicken the cheese and pepperoni.

- Bake an additional 6 minutes or until the chicken reaches an internal temperature of 165 degrees F.

- Serve with steamed broccoli.

Chapter 5:

Dinner Recipes

Broccoli soup

This recipe needs 5 minutes to prepare, 5 minutes to cook and will make 4 servings.

- Protein: 10 grams

- Net Carbs: 5 grams

- Fats: 23 grams

- Calories: 272

What to Use

- Chicken bouillon (.5)

- Pepper (as desired)

- Salt (as desired)

- Onion (.5)

- Broccoli (7 oz.)

- Cheddar cheese (4 oz.)

- Almond milk (.25 c)

- Sour cream (.25 c)

- Cream cheese (.25 c)

- Heavy cream (.25 c)

What to Do

- Remove the florets from the head of broccoli and place them into a bowl. Add a little water to the bowl before microwaving for 3 minutes to steam the broccoli.

- Add all of the liquid ingredients to your blender before adding in the onion, broccoli and cheese. Break the bouillon cube over the top of the rest of the ingredients.

- Blend on the soup setting.

Keto Carnitas

This recipe needs 15 minutes to prepare, 8 hours to cook and will make 16 servings.

- Protein: 8 grams

- Net Carbs: 0grams

- Fats: 19 grams

- Calories: 265

What to Use

- Water (1 c)

- Pepper (as desired)

- Salt (as desired)

- Garlic (4 T minced)

- Chili powder (2 T)

- Thyme (2 T)

- Cumin (2 T)

- Onion (1 large)

- Bacon grease (2 T)

- Pork butt (8 lbs.)

What to Do

- Rub the pork with the seasonings before adding it to the slow cooker.

- Add in the remaining ingredients before letting the slow cooker cook, covered for about 8 hours.

Pizza mushroom

This recipe needs 10 minutes to prepare, 12 minutes to cook and will make 3 servings.

- Protein: 19 grams

- Net Carbs: 4 grams

- Fats: 21 grams

- Calories: 276

What to Use

- Peperoni slice (12)

- Cheddar cheese (1.5 oz.)

- Monterey jack (1.5 oz.)

- Mozzarella (1.5 oz.)

- Spinach (9 leaves)

- Tomato (3 slices)

- Pizza seasoning (3 tsp.)

- Olive oil (to taste)

- Portobello mushrooms (3 large)

What to Do

- Start by making sure your oven is heated to 450F.

- Line a baking sheet using tinfoil and then set the mushrooms onto the baking sheet with the cap facing down before drizzling them in olive oil and seasoning as desired.

- Top with spinach, cheese and tomato before placing in the oven to bake for 6 minutes.

- Remove from the oven, add the pepperoni, and additional seasoning as needed before baking another 6 minutes.

Cheddar biscuit sliders

This recipe needs 15 minutes to prepare, 30 minutes to cook and will make 6 servings.

- Protein: 21 grams

- Net Carbs: 4 grams

- Fats: 43 grams

- Calories: 466

What to Use

- Water (.25 c)

- Heavy cream (.25 c)

- Salt (.5 tsp.)

- Garlic powder (.5 tsp.)

- Cheddar cheese (4 oz.)

- Butter (2 oz. unsalted)

- Carbquik (2 c)

- Hamburger (1 lb.)

- Cheddar cheese (6 slices)

What to Do

- Start by making sure your oven is heated to 450F.

- In a mixing bowl, add in the Carbquick before adding in the butter and mixing until the results start to form a dough.

- Add in the garlic powder, cheese and salt and mix well before adding in the liquid ingredients and mixing to form dough.

- Form the dough into 6 equal sections and place them onto a prepared baking sheet.

- Place the baking sheet in the oven for 8 minutes until the biscuits are golden brown.

- While the biscuits are baking, place the hamburger into a skillet and place the skillet on top of a burner turned to a high/medium heat. As the meat browns, form it into small patties.

- Slice the biscuits in half, and a hamburger patty and slice of cheese to each.

Baked Chicken

This recipe needs 10 minutes to prepare, 20 minutes to cook and will make 4 servings.

- Protein: 63 grams

- Net Carbs: 3 grams

- Fats: 38 grams

- Calories: 527

What to Use

- Cheddar cheese (4 oz.)

- Green onions (3 chopped)

- Ranch dressing (4 oz.)

- Soy sauce (1 oz.)

- Bacon strips (4)

- Chicken breasts (4)

- Coconut oil (2 T)

What to Do

- Place a cast iron skillet on top of a burner turned to a high heat before adding in the coconut oil dand letting it melt.

- Fry the chicken in the pan, flipping regularly for about 10 minutes or until the internal temperature reaches a minimum of 165F.

- While the chicken cooks, add the bacon to a frying pan and place it on the stove over a burner turned to a high/medium heat and let it cook until it is crispy before crumbling it.

- Add the chicken to a baking dish before topping with ranch, soy sauce, ranch, cheese and green onions.

- Broil the baking dish for 3 minutes to give the cheese a chance to brown.

Chicken Curry

This recipe needs 10 minutes to prepare, 30 minutes to cook and will make 6 servings.

- Protein: 38 grams

- Net Carbs: 6 grams

- Fats: 17 grams

- Calories: 349

What to Use

- Coconut oil (3 T)

- Pepper (as desired)

- Salt (as desired)

- Cauliflower (1 head)

- Heavy cream (.5 c)

- Water (1 c)

- Curry paste (1 packet)

- Chicken breast (4)

What to Do

- Add the coconut oil to a large pan before adding in the curry paste and mixing well.

- Add in the water and place the pan on the stove to allow it to simmer a total of 5 minutes.

- Add in the chicken and let it simmer 20 additional minutes.

- While the chicken cooks, turn the cauliflower into cauliflower rice.

- Add the cream in with the chicken and let every cook 5 more minutes.

- Add the cauliflower rice to a bowl and top with chicken curry.

Brussels Sprouts Surprise

This recipe needs 15 minutes to prepare, 30 minutes to cook and will make 12 servings.

- Protein: 13 grams

- Net Carbs: 6 grams

- Fats: 39 grams

- Calories: 350

What to Use

- Butter (2 T melted)

- Almond flour (1 c)

- Parmesan cheese (4 oz. grated)

- Heavy cream (2 c)

- Garlic (2 T minced)

- Thyme (2 tsp.)

- Cheddar cheese (8 oz.)

- Brussels sprouts (2 lb. sliced thin)

What to Do

- Ensure your oven is heated to 350F.

- If you don't want to slice the brussels sprouts by hand, a food processor will also do the trick.

- In a mixing bowl, combine the brussels sprouts with the garlic, thyme and cheese and mix well.

- Add the results to a prepared casserole dish and spread evenly.

- In a separate bowl, combine the butter, parmesan cheese and almond flour and mix until it begins to crumble.

- Add this mixture to the top of the casserole dish and spread evenly.

- Add the dish to the oven for 30 minutes or until the crust has browned and the cheese is bubbling.

Spicy Chicken

This recipe needs 5 minutes to prepare, 35 minutes to cook and will make 4 servings.

- Protein: 44 grams

- Net Carbs: 4 grams

- Fats: 19 grams

- Calories: 281

What to Use

- Pepper (as desired)

- Salt (as desired)

- Onion (1 small chopped)

- Lime juice (3 T)

- Garlic and chili sauce (2 T)

- Chicken thighs (8, skinless, boneless)

What to Do

- Start by making sure your oven is heated to 400F.

- Mix together the salt and pepper as desired before using it to coat the chicken legs thoroughly.

- In a mixing bowl, combine the chili sauce and the lime juice and mix well.

- Add in the chicken and the onion and ensure both are well coated.

- Add all of the ingredients to a large skillet before placing the skillet in the oven for 35 minutes or until the internal temperature of the chicken reaches at least 165F.

Stuffed flank steak

This recipe needs 20 minutes to prepare, 45 minutes to cook and will make 6 servings.

- Protein: 54 grams

- Net Carbs: 3 grams

- Fats: 25 grams

- Calories: 470

What to Use

- Pepper (as desired)

- Salt (as desired)

- Onion powder (.5 tsp.)

- Garlic powder (.5 tsp.)

- Egg yolk (1)

- Almond flour (2 T)

- Bleu cheese (4 oz.)

- Roasted peppers (7 oz. sliced)

- Spinach (16 oz.)

- Flank steak (2)

What to Do

- Ensure you are working with the steak from front to back before beginning to butterfly it, moving from right to left.

- Combine the rest of the ingredients and mix thoroughly in a large mixing bowl.

- Cover the steak in the mixture from the bowl and roll it up as tightly as possible before wrapping it in kitchen twine as tightly as possible.

- Wrap the results in plastic wrap and place the steak in the refrigerator before allowing it to marinate for at least an hour.

- Remove the plastic wrap before placing the steak on a baking sheet and placing the sheet in the oven for 35 minutes.

- Remove the string and broil for 10 minutes, rotating at the halfway point.

- Cover the baking sheet in foil and let it sit for 5 minutes prior to serving.

Keto Burger with Egg

This recipe needs 25 minutes to prepare, 5 minutes to cook and will make 3 servings.

- Protein: 22 grams

- Net Carbs: 1 gram

- Fats: 31 grams

- Calories: 385

What to Use

- Cheddar cheese (8 oz.)

- Worcestershire sauce (to taste)

- Onion powder (.5 tsp.)

- Garlic powder (.5 tsp.)

- Egg (2)

- Ground beef (1.5 lbs.)

- Coconut oil (2 T)

- Bacon (4 strips)

What to Do

- In a mixing bowl, combine the eggs and beef and mix well before adding in the spices and combining thoroughly.

- Break the results down into 1.5 oz. patties before topping each patty with .5 oz. of cheese.

- Combine every 2 patties into a single burger.

- Add the coconut oil to a pan before placing the pan on the stove on top of a burner turned to a high/medium heat. Add in one of the patties and cook each side for approximately 2 minutes or until it reaches your desired level of doneness.

- In a separate frying pan, add in the bacon before placing it on top of a burner turned to a high/medium heat and cook until crispy.

- Top each patty with bacon prior to serving.

Pork Chops

This recipe needs 15 minutes to prepare, 30 minutes to cook and will make 4 servings.

- Protein: 31 grams

- Net Carbs: 3 grams

- Fats: 25 grams

- Calories: 341

What to Use

- Butter (4 T)

- Pepper (as desired)

- Salt (as desired)

- Cumin (1 tsp.)

- Oregano leaves (.5 tsp.)

- Thyme leaves (.5 tsp.)

- Onion powder (1 tsp.)

- Garlic powder (1 tsp.)

- Paprika (1 T)

- Pork chops (4)

What to Do

- In a mixing bowl, combine the paprika, garlic powder, onion powder, thyme leaves, oregano leaves, cumin, salt and pepper in a bowl and mix well.

- Melt the butter in a separate bowl.

- Add some bacon grease to a skillet before placing the skillet on top of a burner turned to a high/medium heat.

- Dip each porkchop in the butter, before coating it thoroughly using the spice and then cooking it for approximately 4 minutes per side in the skillet. The internal temperature of each pork chop should reach around 150F prior to serving.

Keto Quesadilla

This recipe needs 15 minutes to prepare, 9 minutes to cook and will make 4 servings.

- Protein: 16 grams

- Net Carbs: 1 grams

- Fats: 43 grams

- Calories: 462

What to Use

- Eggs (2)

- Jarhlsberg (2 oz.)

- Cheddar cheese (4 oz. shredded)

- Alfredo sauce (.5 c)

- Garlic powder (.5 tsp.)

- Thyme (.5 tsp.)

- Oregano (.5 tsp.)

- Splenda (1.5 tsp.)

- Baking powder (1.5 tsp.)

- Butter (5 T)

- Almond meal (.75 c)

What to Do

- Start by making sure your oven is heated to 350F.

- Add the garlic powder, thyme, oregano, Splenda, baking powder and almond meal together in a mixing bowl and mix well.

- Warm the eggs by placing them in hot water before adding them to the dry mixture before melting the butter and adding it in as well.

- Prepare a pizza pan before adding in the dough and spreading it evenly. Place the pan in the oven and let it cook for 7 minutes.

- Add the shredded cheese and alfredo sauce before placing the pan back in the oven to broil for 2 minutes.

Chapter 6:

Snack Recipes

Spicy Deviled Eggs

This recipe needs 15 minutes to prepare, 15 minutes to cook and will make 6 servings.

- Protein: 15 grams

- Net Carbs: 1.2 grams

- Fats: 42 grams

- Calories: 240

What to Use

- Smoked paprika (.25 tsp.)

- Cream cheese (2 oz. softened)

- Mayonnaise (4 T)

- Bacon (6 slices cooked, crumbled)

- Pickled jalapenos (16 sliced, divided)

- Egg (6)

What to Do

- In a large saucepan, add in the eggs before filling the pan with enough water that the eggs are submerged under 1 inch of water.

- Add the pan to the stove over a saucepan turned to a high heat. After the water boils, remove the pan from the stove and let the contents cool for 12 minutes.

- Peel the eggs and cut them in half vertically.

- Add the yolks to a mixing bowl and mash well. Add in the jalapenos, cream cheese, mayonnaise and bacon.

- Add the results to each of the egg halves, chill, serve and enjoy.

Bacon wrapped mozzarella

This recipe needs 10 minutes to prepare, 3 minutes to cook and will make 2 servings.

- Protein: 3 grams

- Net Carbs: .5 grams

- Fats: 32 grams

- Calories: 200

What to Use

- Pizza sauce (as needed)

- Coconut Oil (1 cup)

- Bacon (2 slices)

- Cheese stick (1 halved)

What to Do

- Ensure your deep fryer is preheated to 350 degrees F.

- Wrap each mozzarella stick half in bacon and secure it with the help of a toothpick.

- Fry the mozzarella stick halves for 3 minutes.

- Serve with marinara sauce.

Bacon onion butter

This recipe needs 15 minutes to prepare, 5 minutes to cook and will make 8 servings (1 serving is 1 T butter).

- Protein: 1 grams

- Net Carbs: 1.1 grams

- Fats: 36 grams

- Calories: 151

What to Use

- Black pepper (as needed)

- Salt (as needed)

- Worcestershire sauce (to taste)

- Spicy mustard (to taste)

- Onion (1.5 sliced, diced)

- Bacon (4 strips)

- Butter (9 T)

What to Do

- Add 1 T of butter to a skillet before placing the skillet above a burner set to a medium heat.

- Add in the bacon, then the onion and let the onion fry until the bacon has cooked.

- Combine the butter, bacon, onions and desired seasoning together in a large mixing bowl and mix extremely well.

- Refrigerate prior to use.

Bacon and cauliflower bites

This recipe needs 15 minutes to prepare, 30 minutes to cook and will make 10 servings.

- Protein: 2 grams

- Net Carbs: 1.2 grams

- Fats: 26 grams

- Calories: 201

What to Use

- Cauliflower rice (5 c)

- Cream cheese (8 oz. softened)

- Goat cheese (4 oz.)

- Black pepper (as needed)

- Salt (as needed)

- Garlic Powder (1 teaspoon)

- Onion powder (1 teaspoon)

- Italian seasoning (1 teaspoon divided)

- Garlic (3 cloves minced)

- Panko (.5 cups)

- Crushed pork rinds (1 cup)

- White cheddar cheese (.5 cups)

- Sharp cheddar cheese (.5 cups)

- Parmesan cheese (1.5 cups divided)

What to Do

- Turn the cauliflower into rice by processing it using a food processor.

- Mix together the salt, pepper, .5 teaspoon Italian seasoning, minced garlic, .5 cups grated parmesan cheese, white cedar cheese, sharp cheddar cheese, goat cheese, cream cheese, bacon and cauliflower in a mixing bowl. Place the bowl in the refrigerator for 60 minutes.

- In a separate bowl, combine the Italian seasoning, garlic powder, onion powder, panko, parmesan cheese and pork rinds and mix well.

- Once it has cooled, roll the contents of the first bowl into balls before coating with the mixture in the second bowl.

- About roughly 1 inch of oil to a large frying pan before placing it on the stove above a burner turned to a high/medium heat. Once the oil heats up, add in 5 of the balls at a time and fry for 6 minutes so they are golden brown.

Olive and tomato fat bomb

This recipe needs 10 minutes to prepare, 35 minutes to harden and will make 5 servings.

- Protein: 3.7 grams

- Net Carbs: 1.7 grams

- Fats: 17.1 grams

- Calories: 164

What to Use

- Parmesan cheese (5 T grated)

- Salt (.25 tsp.)

- Black pepper (to taste)

- Garlic (2 cloves crushed)

- Kalamata olives (4 pitted)

- Sun-dried tomatoes (4 pieces drained)

- Oregano (2 T chopped)

- Thyme (2 T chopped)

- Basil (2 T chopped)

- Butter (.25 c)

- Cream cheese (.5 c)

What to Do

- Chop the butter and add it to a small mixing bowl with the cream cheese and leave them both to soften for about 30 minutes. Mash together and mix well to combine.

- Add in the Kalamata olives and sun-dried tomatoes and mix well before adding in the herbs and seasonings. Combine thoroughly before placing the mixing bowl in the refrigerator to allow the results to solidify.

- Once it has solidified, form the mixture into a total of 5 balls using an ice cream scoop. Roll each of the finished balls into the parmesan cheese before plating.

- Extras can be stored in the refrigerator in an air-tight container for up to 7 days.

Breakfast fat bomb

This recipe needs 15 minutes active preparation, 30 minutes total and will make 6 servings.

- Protein: .2 grams

- Net Carbs: .2 grams

- Fats: 18.4 grams

- Calories: 185

What to Use

- Bacon (4 slices)

- Salt (.25 tsp.)

- Black pepper (to taste)

- Keto mayo (2 T)

- Ghee (.25 c)

- Eggs (2 large)

What to Do

- Start by making sure your oven is heated to 375F.

- Prepare a baking tray by lining it with parchment paper before placing the bacon strips on top, taking care to ensure that they do not overlap.

- Place the tray in the oven and let it cook for about 10 minutes until crispy. Remove the bacon from the oven and let it cool.

- In a small pot, place the eggs and add cold water until the eggs are completely covered by roughly 1 inch of water. Add the pot to the stove above a boiler turned to a high/medium heat and let the water boil.

- After the water has boiled, remove the pot from the stove and let it cool for roughly 10 minutes and then drain the pot.

- Fill a large bowl with cold water and dunk the eggs briefly into it to make them easier to peel before cutting them into quarters.

- In a small mixing bowl, slice the butter and add in the eggs before mashing them using fork before adding in the seasonings as well as the mayo and mixing well. Add in the bacon grease and combine thoroughly.

- Add the results to the refrigerator and let them chill for approximately 20 minutes until they can be worked with easily.

- Crumble the bacon into a small bowl, the bomb mixture should be enough for 6 balls, roll them up and then roll each in bacon before returning them to the refrigerator to harden prior to serving.

Guacamole fat bomb

This recipe needs 10 minutes active preparation, 45 minutes total and will make 6 servings.

- Protein: 3.4 grams

- Net Carbs: 2.7 grams

- Fats: 15.2 grams

- Calories: 156

What to Use

- Bacon (4 slices)

- Cilantro (2 T)

- Salt (.25 tsp.)

- Black pepper (to taste)

- Lime juice (1 T)

- White onion (.5 Diced)

- Chili pepper (1 chopped fine)

- Garlic (2 cloves crushed)

- Ghee (.25 c)

- Avocado (.5 large)

What to Do

- Start by making sure your oven is heated to 375F.

- Prepare a baking tray by lining it with parchment paper before placing the bacon strips on top, taking care to ensure that they do not overlap.

- Place the tray in the oven and let it cook for about 10 minutes until crispy. Remove the bacon from the oven and let it cool.

- Peel the avocado, cut it in half and remove the seed before adding it to a mixing bowl. Add in the lime juice, cilantro, garlic, pepper but and any seasonings and mash the results until everything is thoroughly combined. Mix in the onion.

- Add in the bacon grease and combine thoroughly. Cover the bowl in tinfoil and let it chill in the refrigerator for 30 minutes.

- Crumble the bacon into a small bowl, the bomb mixture should be enough for 6 balls, roll them up and then roll each in bacon before returning them to the refrigerator to harden prior to serving.

Iced bulletproof coffee

This recipe needs 5 minutes active preparation and will make 1 serving.

- Protein: 0 grams

- Net Carbs: 0 grams

- Fats: 10 grams

- Calories: 89

What to Use

- Coffee (2 c)

- Coconut cream (1 tsp.)

- Ghee (1 tsp.)

- Coconut oil (1 tsp.)

- Ice cubes (4)

What to Do

- Add all of the ingredients to a blender and blend until your desired consistency is achieved.

- Drink promptly for best results.

Bacon and butter fat bomb

This recipe needs 2 minutes active preparation, and will make 3 servings.

- Protein: 9 grams

- Net Carbs:.7 grams

- Fats: 17 grams

- Calories: 158

What to Use

- Pecan halves (2 toasted, chopped)

- Granulated garlic (1 pinch)

- Kerrygold butter (1 T)

- Bacon (1 large, thick slice cooked)

What to Do

- Take the piece of and split it into three parts, add 1 T butter to each before topping with a piece of pecan.

Fishy fat bomb

This recipe needs 10 minutes active preparation, 60 minutes total and will make 6 servings.

- Protein: 3.2 grams

- Net Carbs: .8 grams

- Fats: 15.7 grams

- Calories: 147

What to Use

- Salt (1 pinch)

- Dill (2 T chopped)

- Lemon juice (1 T)

- Smoked salmon (1.8 oz.)

- Ghee (.3 c)

- Cream cheese (.5 c)

What to Do

- Add the smoked salmon, butter and cream cheese to a food processor along with the dill and lemon juice and pulse generously.

- Prepare a serving tray by covering it with parchment paper before spooning out the salmon mixture in 2.5 T dollops.

- Top with additional dill and let chill in the refrigerator for at least 60 minutes prior to serving.

Meatloaf fat bomb

This recipe needs 15 minutes active preparation, 30 minutes total and will make 6 servings.

- Protein: .2 grams

- Net Carbs: .2 grams

- Fats: 18.4 grams

- Calories: 185

What to Use

- Bacon (8 strips + .5 lb. chunked)

- Coconut milk (.25 c)

- Garlic (2 cloves crushed)

- Chives (.3 c minced)

- Salt (as desired)

- Pepper (as desired)

- Ground beef (1 lb.)

What to Do

- Start by making sure your oven is heated to 400F.

- In a mixing bowl, combine the chunks of bacon, coconut milk and beef and mix thoroughly before seasoning as desired.

- Prepare a muffin tin before adding a slice of bacon to each of them and filling the remaining space with meat mixture.

- Place the tin in the oven for 30 minutes.

- Let cool 5 minutes prior to serving.

Chapter 7:

Dessert Recipes

Keto Fudge

This recipe needs 10 minutes to prepare, 60 minutes to freeze and will make 12 servings.

- Protein: 3 grams

- Net Carbs: 0.6 grams

- Fats: 29 grams

- Calories: 241

What to Use

- Clarified butter (.6 c melted)

- Coconut oil (.6 c melted)

- Keto maple syrup (1 T)

- Vanilla pod (1)

What to Do

- Combine all of the ingredients together in a food processor and process well.

- Pour the results into a glass dish and let it freeze for 60 minutes prior to cutting.

Keto Chocolate

This recipe needs 15 minutes to prepare, 40 minutes to freeze and will make 12 servings.

- Protein: 3 grams

- Net Carbs: 1.3 grams

- Fats: 34.3 grams

- Calories: 121

What to Use

- Shredded coconut (2 cups)

- Coconut oil (.25 cups)

- Chocolate unsweetened (4 squares)

- Coconut oil (1.25 Tablespoons)

- Stevia (24 liquid drops)

What to Do

- Melt the coconut oil before adding it, half of the stevia and the other coconut to a food process and pulse repeatedly.

- Pour the contents of the food processor into a silicone pan and let it freeze in the freezer.

- Add the rest of the coconut oil as well as the chocolate to another bowl and melt them together before adding in the rest of the stevia and mixing well.

- Add the chocolate to the rest of the frozen ingredients and let it freeze for at least 30 minutes before cutting into squares.

Coconut and cinnamon fat bomb

This recipe needs 90 minutes to prepare, 5 minutes to cook and will make 12 servings.

- Protein: 2.3 grams

- Net Carbs: 2 grams

- Fats: 19 grams

- Calories: 201

What to Use

- Coconut butter (1.25 cups)

- Coconut milk (.75 cups)

- Vanilla extract (1.25 teaspoons)

- Nutmeg (.25 teaspoons)

- Cinnamon (.75 teaspoons)

- Powdered stevia (1 teaspoon)

- Coconut (1 cup shredded)

What to Do

- In a double broiler, add the coconut milk, coconut butter, nutmeg, vanilla extract, stevia and cinnamon before adding the double broiler to the stove on top of a burner set to medium.

- Stir well as the ingredients melt.

- After mixing well, add the result to a bowl and let the bowl chill for half an hour.

- Shape the contents of the bowl into balls and coat the balls in the coconut.

- Let them harden for 60 minutes for best results.

Peanut butter fudge

This recipe needs 15 minutes active preparation, 45 minutes total and will make 20 servings.

- Protein: 37 grams

- Net Carbs: 4.7 grams

- Fats: 52.5 grams

- Calories: 107

What to Use

- Walnuts (.25 c chopped)

- Salt (1 dash)

- Cocoa powder (.3 c)

- Vanilla whey protein powder (1 scoop)

- Stevia (to taste)

- Vanilla extract (.5 tsp.)

- Cream cheese (2 oz.)

- Peanut butter (.5 c)

- Coconut oil (.5 c)

What to Do

- Line a baking dish (5x7) using parchment paper, taking care to leave extra space on the side to make it easier to remove later.

- Add the peanut butter and the regular butter to a saucepan before placing it on a burner turned to a low heat until it can be easily mixed together.

- In another bowl, add in the cream cheese and beat it before adding in the butter and peanut butter mixture and blending well. Mix in the stevia as well as the vanilla.

- In a third bowl, mix together the salt, cocoa powder and whey protein powder. Mix together the two bowls and combine thoroughly before mixing in the nuts.

- Spread the mixture into the prepared pan and freeze for 30 minutes prior to cutting.

Coconut and ginger fat bomb

This recipe needs 5 minutes active preparation, 5 minutes total and will make 10 servings.

- Protein: .5 grams

- Net Carbs: 2.2 grams

- Fats: 12.5 grams

- Calories: 121

What to Use

- Ginger (1 tsp.)

- Stevia (1 tsp.)

- Shredded coconut (25 g)

- Coconut oil (75 g)

- Coconut butter (75 g softened)

What to Do

- Add all of the ingredients to a blender and blend well.

- Pour the results into a silicon mold and let it freeze prior to serving.

Lemon Fat bomb

This recipe needs 5 minutes active preparation, 40 minutes total and will make 16 servings.

- Protein: .7 grams

- Net Carbs: .8 grams

- Fats: 11.9 grams

- Calories: 112

What to Use

- Stevia (to taste)

- Sea salt (1 pinch)

- Lemon zest (2 T)

- Coconut oil (.25 c)

- Coconut butter (7.1 oz. softened)

What to Do

- Combine all of the ingredients in a mixing bowl. Take special care to ensure that both the stevia and lemon zest are evenly distributed.

- Fill a silicon candy model with 1 T of the mixture per square and let them freeze prior to serving.

Vanilla nut fat bomb

This recipe needs 10 minutes active preparation, 40 minutes total and will make 14 servings.

- Protein: .8 grams

- Net Carbs: .6 grams

- Fats: 14.4 grams

- Calories: 132

What to Use

- Stevia (to taste)

- Erythritol (2 T)

- Vanilla bean (1 crushed)

- Ghee (.25 c)

- Coconut oil (.25 c)

- Macadamia nuts (1 c unsalted)

What to Do

- Add the macadamia nuts to a food processor and process well.

- Leave the ghee out on the counter until it reaches room temperature before mixing it together with the coconut oil.

- Add in the vanilla bean, stevia and erythritol and mix well.

- Add the results to a pair of ice cube trays so that 1.5 T is used per serving.

- Freeze prior to serving.

Spicy chocolate fat bombs

This recipe needs 10 minutes active preparation, 60 minutes total and will make 10 servings.

- Protein: 1.8 grams

- Net Carbs: 1.1 grams

- Fats: 9.4 grams

- Calories: 50

What to Use

- Stevia (to taste)

- Erythritol (2 T)

- Cayenne pepper (.25 tsp.)

- Cinnamon (1 tsp.)

- Vanilla extract (1 tsp.)

- Cocoa powder (2 T unsweetened)

- Coconut milk (1 cup)

What to Do

- Place the coconut milk in a microwave safe container and warm it for 35 seconds in the microwave.

- Add in all of the remaining ingredients and mix well.

- Add 1 T of the mixture to a full set of ice cube trays and let it freeze prior to serving.

Raspberry chocolate fat bomb

This recipe needs 20 minutes active preparation, 90 minutes total and will make 14 servings.

- Protein: 2.2 grams

- Net Carbs: 2.6 grams

- Fats: 17.1 grams

- Calories: 164

What to Use

- Stevia (to taste)

- Erythritol (.5 c powdered)

- Vanilla extract (1 tsp.)

- Cacao powder (.3 c)

- Dark chocolate (4.2 oz.)

- Coconut oil (3 T)

- Cocoa butter (.5 c)

- Almonds (1 oz. roasted)

- 1.5 c raspberries)

What to Do

- Stick and almond inside of each raspberry and freeze them for 60 minutes.

- In a glass bowl, combine the unsweetened chocolate, coconut oil and cocoa butter. Place the bowl on top of a pan full of water and place the pan on top of a burner turned to a high heat.

- Stir continuously while the ingredients melt and combine thoroughly.

- Add in the remaining dry ingredients and mix well.

- Dip each raspberry in the chocolate before placing them on a lined serving sheet.

- Place the sheet in the refrigerator to chill prior to serving.

Blueberry fat bomb

This recipe needs 5 minutes active preparation, 40 minutes total and will make 16 servings.

- Protein: 1 gram

- Net Carbs: 1 gram

- Fats: 13 grams

- Calories: 116

What to Use

- Stevia (to taste)

- Coconut cream (.25 c)

- Cream cheese (4 oz. softened)

- Coconut oil (.75 c)

- Butter (4 oz.)

- Blueberries (1 c)

What to Do

- Add the cream cheese, coconut cream and berries into a food processor and process well.

- Add the coconut oil and the butter to a saucepan before placing the pan on a burner turned to a low heat and mix well as the butter melts. Let cool 5 minutes prior to adding to the food processor.

- Process well before adding in the stevia and process again.

- Add the result to a pair of ice cube trays in 1 T serving sizes. Freeze 40 minutes prior to serving.

Strawberry fat bomb

This recipe needs 10 minutes active preparation, 40 minutes total and will make 12 servings.

- Protein: .5 grams

- Net Carbs: .1 grams

- Fats: 10 grams

- Calories: 90

What to Use

- Stevia (to taste)

- Strawberries (3 diced)

- heavy cream (2 oz.)

- coconut oil (4 T)

- butter (4 T)

What to Do

- In an emersion blender, combine the heavy cream and the strawberries and blend well.

- Add the butter to a microwave safe container and microwave if for 30 seconds before mixing in the stevia.

- Add all of the remaining ingredients to the blender and blend well.

- Add the result to a pair of ice cube trays in 1 T serving sizes. Freeze 40 minutes prior to serving.

Conclusion

Thank you for making it through to the end of *The Essential Ketogenic Cookbook: 55 Ketogenic Diet Recipes*, let's hope it was informative and able to provide you with all of the tools you need to achieve your weight loss goals, whatever it is that they may be. Just because you've finished this book doesn't mean you have run out of new ketogenic meal ideas to try, what you have read should give you a great template to build from when it comes to finding your footing with your new ketogenic diet.

When first committing to the keto diet full time, it is important to not underestimate just how difficult the transition will be, as doing so will only make it all the harder. As such, in order to find the success, you seek you are going to need to go into the process fully committing to the change, which means vowing to follow through no matter how difficult things get in the interim. Remember, forewarned is forearmed and if you go in committed to seeing it through no matter what, then your odds of succeeding increase dramatically.

Making it through to the other side is only half the battle, however, as the ketogenic diet is a lifestyle, not something you are going to switch to and then abandon a few months down the line. Only by committing to the long-term will you be able to truly take advantage of all the health and weight loss benefits that the keto lifestyle has to offer. Remember, becoming keto is a marathon, not a sprint, slow and steady wins the race.

Note From The Author

Thank you for reading this book! If you enjoyed it, please consider posting an honest review on Amazon. Reviews are very important to us independent Amazon authors, and each one we get matters. It would be highly appreciated if you write your own review. Thanks again for reading!